The Mediterranean Meat Cooking Guide

A Complete Collection of Mediterranean Recipes to
Enjoy Meat and Boost Your Diet

Raymond Morton

Table of contents

Chicken Wings Mix

Prep time: 10 minutes I **Cooking time:** 50 minutes I
Servings: 4

Ingredients:

- 2 tablespoons olive oil
- 1 yellow onion, chopped
- 2 tablespoons olive oil
- A pinch of salt and black pepper
- 2 pounds chicken wings
- ½ pound sweet potatoes, peeled and cut into wedges
- ½ cup coconut cream
- 1 and ½ tablespoons tarragon, chopped

Directions:

1. Heat up a pan with the oil over medium-high heat, add the onion and sauté for 5 minutes.
2. Add the meat and cook for 5 minutes more.
3. Add the rest of the ingredients, toss, introduce in the oven and bake at 360 degrees F for 40 minutes.
4. Divide the mix between plates and serve.

Nutrition info per serving: calories 698, fat 38.1, fiber 3.6, carbs 20.1, protein 67.5

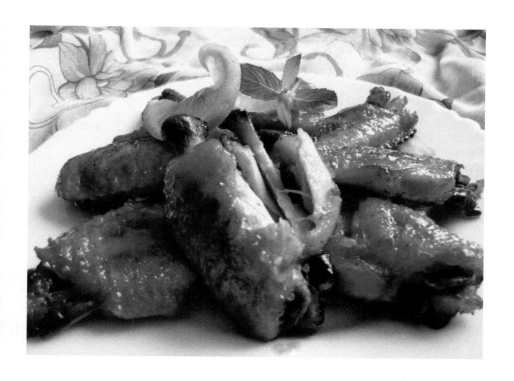

Walnuts Chives Chicken Mix

Prep time: 10 minutes I **Cooking time:** 45 minutes I
Servings: 4

Ingredients:

- 1 yellow onion, chopped
- 2 tablespoons olive oil
- 3 garlic cloves, minced
- 1 pound chicken thighs, skinless, boneless
- ½ cup chicken stock
- 2 bay leaves
- 3 tablespoons walnuts, chopped
- A pinch of salt and black pepper
- 2 tablespoons chives, chopped

Directions:

1. Heat up a pan with the oil over medium-high heat, add the onion and the garlic and sauté for 5 minutes.
2. Add the chicken and brown for 5 minutes more.
3. Add the rest of the ingredients, stir, cook over medium heat for 30 minutes more, divide between plates and serve.

Nutrition info per serving: calories 229, fat 7, fiber 7, carbs 15, protein 18

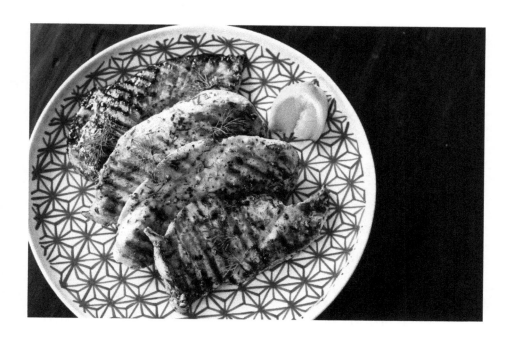

Chicken with Basil Beans

Prep time: 5 minutes I **Cooking time:** 8 hours I
Servings: 4

Ingredients:

- 1 yellow onion, chopped
- 2 carrots, sliced
- 2 garlic cloves, minced
- 2 pounds chicken breast, skinless, boneless and cubed
- 10 ounces kidney beans, cooked
- 1 teaspoon cumin, ground
- ½ teaspoon basil, dried
- A pinch of salt and black pepper
- 1 tablespoon oregano, chopped

Directions:

1. In a slow cooker, combine chicken with the onion, the carrots, the garlic and the other ingredients, toss, put the lid on and cook on Low for 8 hours.
2. Divide the mix between plates and serve.

Nutrition info per serving: calories 299, fat 3, fiber 7, carbs 13, protein 19

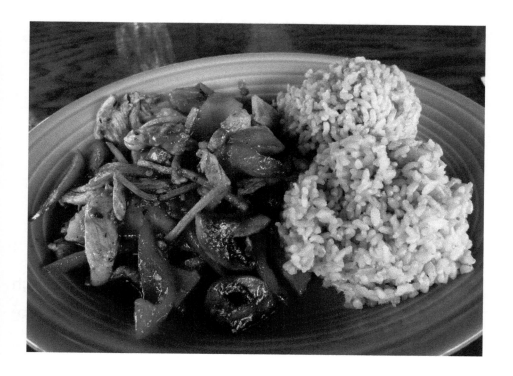

Chicken and Green Beans Mix

Prep time: 5 minutes I **Cooking time:** 30 minutes I
Servings: 4

Ingredients:

- 1 cup chicken stock
- 2 tablespoons olive oil
- 1 pound chicken thighs, bone-in and skin-on
- A pinch of salt and black pepper
- 1 yellow onion, chopped
- 2 cups green beans, trimmed and halved
- ¼ cup basil, chopped
- 2 tablespoons capers
- 1 tablespoon lemon juice

Directions:

1. Heat up a pan with the oil over medium-high heat, add the onion and the chicken and sauté for 5 minutes.

Add the rest of the ingredients, toss, cook over medium heat for 25 minutes more, divide between plates and serve.

Nutrition info per serving: calories 300, fat 5, fiber 7, carbs 11, protein 16

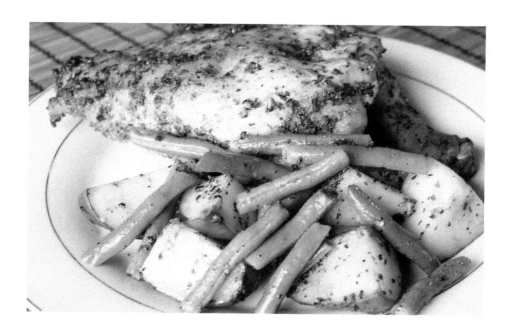

Chicken with Beets

Prep time: 10 minutes I **Cooking time:** 40 minutes I
Servings: 4

Ingredients:

- 1 pound chicken breast, skinless, boneless and sliced
- A pinch of salt and black pepper
- 1 teaspoon sweet paprika
- 1 yellow onion, chopped
- 1 teaspoon coriander, ground
- 2 tablespoons avocado oil
- Juice of 1 lemon
- 4 garlic cloves, minced
- 1 cup Brussels sprouts, trimmed and halved
- 2 beets, peeled and cubed
- 1 tablespoon rosemary, chopped

Directions:

1. Heat up a pan with the oil over medium-high heat, add the onion and the garlic and sauté for 5 minutes.
2. Add the meat and brown for 5 minutes more.

3. Add the rest of the ingredients, toss, cook over medium heat for 30 minutes more, divide between plates and serve.

Nutrition info per serving: calories 297, fat 7, fiber 6, carbs 11, protein 19

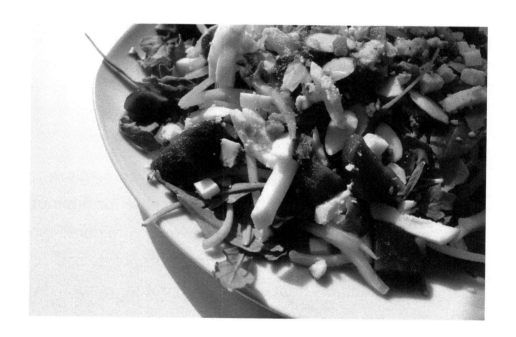

Chicken with Chives Grapes

Prep time: 10 minutes I **Cooking time:** 40 minutes I
Servings: 4

Ingredients:

- 1 cup grapes, halved
- 2 pounds chicken breast, skinless, boneless and cubed
- 2 teaspoons curry powder
- 2 tablespoons avocado oil
- 4 scallions, chopped
- A pinch of salt and black pepper
- 1 tablespoon chives, chopped

Directions:

1. Heat up a pan with the oil over medium-high heat, add the scallions and sauté for 5 minutes.
2. Add the chicken and brown for 5 minutes more.
3. Add the rest of the ingredients, toss, cook over medium heat for 30 minutes more, divide between plates and serve.

Nutrition info per serving: calories 222, fat 5, fiber 7, carbs 14, protein 17

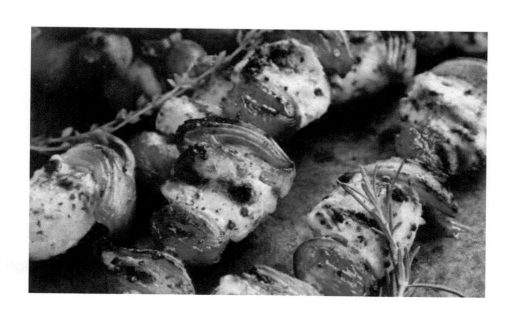

Chicken with Bok Choy

Prep time: 10 minutes I **Cooking time:** 40 minutes I
Servings: 4

Ingredients:

- 2 pounds chicken breast, skinless, boneless and cubed
- 1 cup bok choy, torn
- 2 tablespoons olive oil
- 4 garlic cloves, minced
- A pinch of salt and black pepper
- Cooking spray
- ½ cup pecans, roasted
- 1 tablespoon chives, chopped

Directions:

1. Heat up a pan with the oil over medium-high heat, add the garlic and sauté for 2 minutes.
2. Add the meat and brown for 5 minutes more.
3. Add the rest of the ingredients, toss, cook over medium heat for 33 minutes more, divide between plates and serve.

Nutrition info per serving: calories 300, fat 12, fiber 7, carbs 15, protein 18

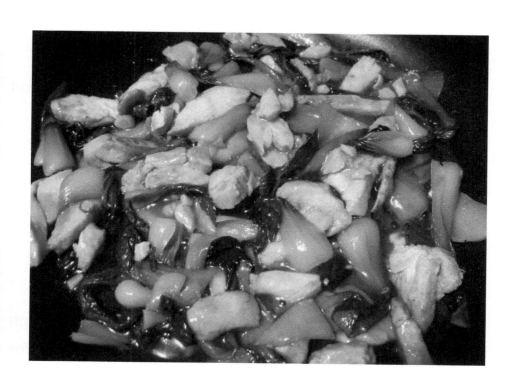

Turkey and Tomatoes

Prep time: 10 minutes I **Cooking time:** 40 minutes I
Servings: 4

Ingredients:

- 1 yellow onion, chopped
- 2 garlic cloves, minced
- 1 pound turkey breast, skinless, boneless and cut into strips
- 1 cup tomatoes, roughly cubed
- 2 tablespoons olive oil
- 1 tablespoon tarragon, chopped
- A pinch of salt and black pepper
- 1 teaspoon smoked paprika

Directions:

1. Heat up a pan with the oil over medium-high heat, add the onion and the garlic and sauté for 5 minutes.
2. Add the meat and brown for 5 minutes more.
3. Add the remaining ingredients, toss, cook over medium for 30 minutes more, divide between plates and serve.

Nutrition info per serving: calories 298, fat 8, fiber 4, carbs 14, protein 15

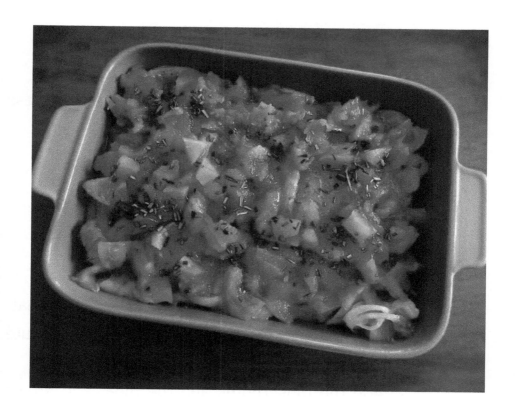

Chicken and Mushrooms

Prep time: 10 minutes I **Cooking time:** 40 minutes I
Servings: 4

Ingredients:

- 2 tablespoons olive oil
- 1 yellow onion, chopped
- ½ pounds Bella mushrooms, sliced
- 2 pounds chicken thighs, boneless and skinless
- 3 carrots, sliced
- 2 celery stalks, chopped
- ½ cup coconut cream
- 1 tablespoon thyme, chopped
- 1 tablespoon cilantro, chopped

Directions:

1. Heat up a pan with the oil over medium heat, add the onion, carrots and the celery and sauté for 5 minutes.
2. Add the mushrooms and the meat and brown for 5 minutes more.
3. Add the rest of the ingredients, toss, cook over medium heat for 30 minutes more, divide between plates and serve.

Nutrition info per serving: calories 300, fat 6, fiber 7, carbs 15, protein 16

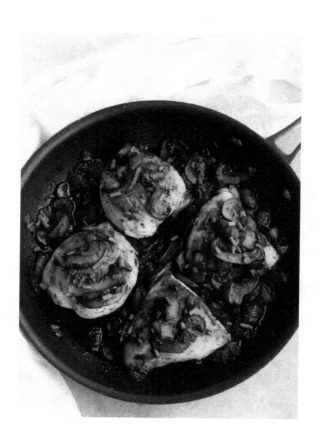

Chicken with Balsamic Plums

Prep time: 10 minutes I **Cooking time:** 45 minutes I
Servings: 4

Ingredients:

- 2 pounds chicken breast, skinless, boneless and cubed
- 4 scallions, chopped
- 2 tablespoons olive oil
- A pinch of salt and black pepper
- 1 teaspoon ginger, grated
- 4 garlic cloves, minced
- 2 cups plums, pitted and halved
- 1 tablespoon balsamic vinegar
- 2 tablespoons cilantro, chopped

Directions:

1. Heat up a pan with the oil over medium heat, add the scallions, ginger and the garlic and sauté for 5 minutes.
2. Add the chicken and brown for 5 minutes more.
3. Add the plums and the rest of the ingredients, toss, cook over medium heat for 35 minutes more, divide between plates and serve.

Nutrition info per serving: calories 280, fat 8, fiber 4, carbs 12, protein 17

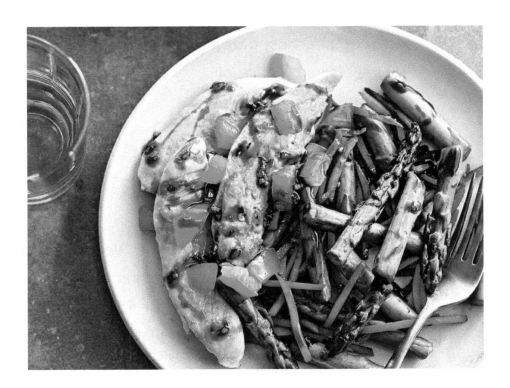

Turkey with Apples

Prep time: 10 minutes I **Cooking time:** 45 minutes I
Servings: 4

Ingredients:

- 2 pound turkey breast, skinless, boneless and sliced
- 1 green apple, cored and cut into wedges
- 1 cup peaches, pitted and cubed
- 1 tablespoon olive oil
- 2 green chilies, chopped
- A pinch of black pepper
- 1 teaspoon chili powder
- 1 tablespoon lime juice

Directions:

1. In a roasting pan, combine the turkey with the apple, peaches and the other ingredients, toss and bake at 390 degrees F for 45 minutes.
2. Divide everything between plates and serve.

Nutrition info per serving: calories 314, fat 7.6, fiber 3.3, carbs 22.1, protein 39.3

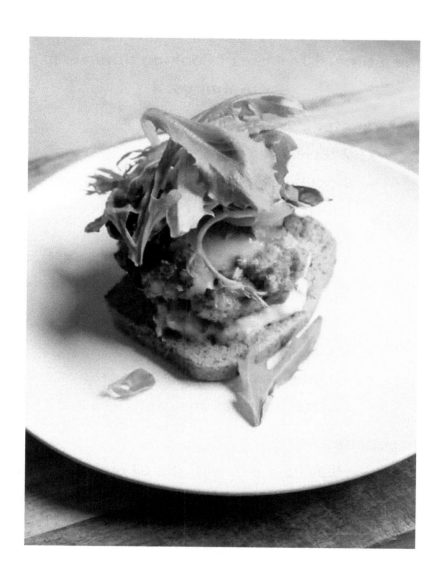

Chicken with Chili Quinoa

Prep time: 10 minutes I **Cooking time:** 40 minutes I
Servings: 4

Ingredients:

- 2 tablespoons avocado oil
- 1 pound chicken breast, skinless, boneless and cubed
- A pinch of salt and black pepper
- 1 cup quinoa
- ½ teaspoon chili powder
- ½ teaspoon cumin, ground
- 3 cups chicken stock
- 4 green onions, chopped
- 1 tablespoon sesame seeds, toasted

Directions:

1. Heat up a pan with the oil over medium heat, add the green onions and the chicken and brown for 5 minutes.
2. Add the rest of the ingredients, toss, bring to a simmer and cook over medium heat for 35 minutes more.

3. Divide everything between plates and serve.

Nutrition info per serving: calories 322, fat 8, fiber 4.1, carbs 30.2, protein 31.4

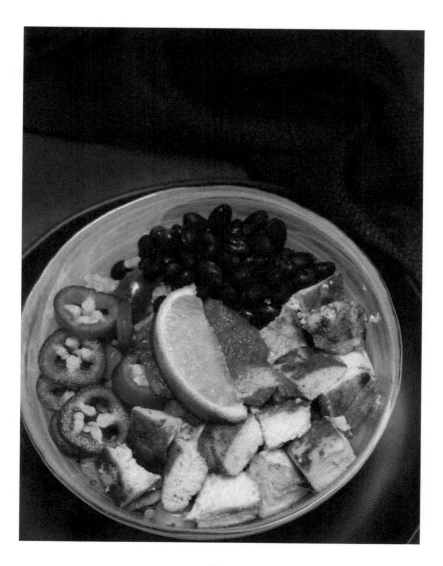

Chicken with Berry Sauce

Prep time: 10 minutes I **Cooking time:** 35 minutes I
Servings: 4

Ingredients:

- 4 scallions, chopped
- 2 tablespoons avocado oil
- 2 pounds chicken breasts, skinless, boneless and sliced
- 2 tablespoons balsamic vinegar
- 1 cup chicken stock
- 2 cups raspberries
- A pinch of salt and black pepper
- 1 tablespoon cilantro, chopped

Directions:

1. Heat up a pan with the oil over medium-high heat, add the scallions and the meat and brown for 5 minutes.
2. Add the rest of the ingredients, toss, cook over medium heat for 30 minutes more, divide between plates and serve.

Nutrition info per serving: calories 481, fat 18.3, fiber 4.7, carbs 9.1, protein 66.9

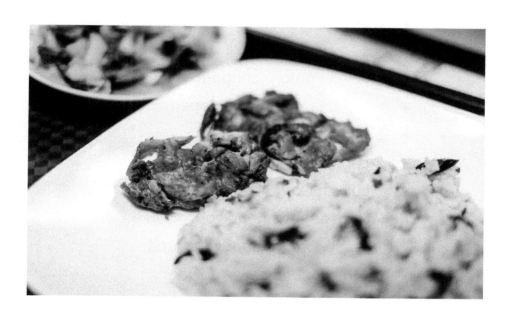

Coriander Turkey Curry

Prep time: 10 minutes I **Cooking time:** 40 minutes I
Servings: 4

Ingredients:

- 1 pound turkey breast, boneless, skinless and cubed
- 1 yellow onion, chopped
- 1 red bell pepper, chopped
- 2 tablespoons avocado oil
- 1 cup coconut cream
- 1 cup chicken stock
- ½ teaspoon chili powder
- 1 teaspoon coriander, ground
- 3 tablespoons curry powder
- 2 tablespoons cilantro, chopped
- A pinch of salt and black pepper

Directions:

1. Heat up a pan with the oil over medium-high heat, add the onion and the turkey meat and brown for 5 minutes.
2. Add the bell pepper and the other ingredients, toss, cook over medium heat for 35 minutes more, divide into bowls and serve.

Nutrition info per serving: calories 280, fat 13, fiber 7, carbs 8, protein 15

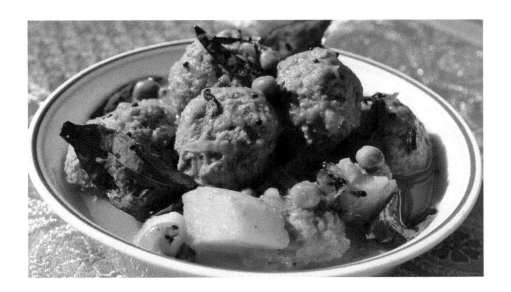

Turmeric Chicken and Avocado

Prep time: 10 minutes I **Cooking time:** 35 minutes I
Servings: 4

Ingredients:

- 4 garlic cloves, minced
- 4 scallions, chopped
- 2 pounds chicken thighs, skinless and boneless
- 2 tablespoons olive oil
- 1 avocado, peeled, pitted and sliced
- 1 teaspoon turmeric powder
- A pinch of salt and black pepper
- 1 teaspoon red chili flakes

Directions:

1. Heat up a pan with the oil over medium-high heat, add the scallions and the garlic and sauté for 5 minutes.
2. Add the meat and brown for 5 minutes more.
3. Add the rest of the ingredients, toss, cook over medium heat for 25 minutes more, divide between plates and serve.

Nutrition info per serving: calories 200, fat 10, fiber 1, carbs 12, protein 24

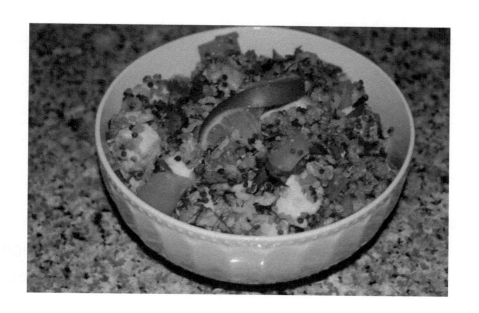

Ginger Chicken Thighs

Prep time: 5 minutes I **Cooking time:** 40 minutes I
Servings: 4

Ingredients:

- 2 pounds chicken thighs, boneless, skinless
- 2 tablespoons olive oil
- 4 scallions, chopped
- 2 sweet potatoes, peeled and cut into wedges
- 1 tablespoon lemon juice
- 1 teaspoon coriander, ground
- A pinch of salt and black pepper
- 1 tablespoon ginger, minced
- 1 tablespoon rosemary, chopped

Directions:

1. Heat up a pan with the oil over medium-high heat, add the scallions, ginger and the meat and brown for 10 minutes stirring often.
2. Add the rest of the ingredients, toss, cook over medium heat for 30 minutes more, divide between plates and serve.

Nutrition info per serving: calories 210, fat 8, fiber 4, carbs 12, protein 17

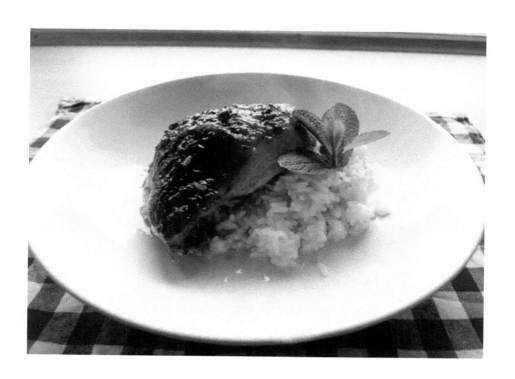

Hot Turkey

Prep time: 10 minutes I **Cooking time:** 1 hour I
Servings: 4

Ingredients:

- 2 tablespoons avocado oil
- 2 pounds turkey breast, skinless, boneless and cubed
- 1 green bell pepper, chopped
- 1 orange bell pepper, chopped
- 2 garlic cloves, minced
- 3 scallions, chopped
- 1 red chili, chopped
- ½ teaspoon chili flakes, crushed
- 1 tablespoon chili powder
- 15 ounces tomatoes, chopped
- 1 cup veggie stock
- A pinch of salt and black pepper

Directions:

1. Heat up a pan with the oil over medium heat, add the scallions and the garlic and sauté for 5 minutes.
2. Add the meat and brown for 5 minutes more.

3. Add the bell peppers and the other ingredients, toss, cook over medium heat for 50 minutes more, divide into bowls and serve.

Nutrition info per serving: calories 220, fat 8, fiber 4, carbs 14, protein 13

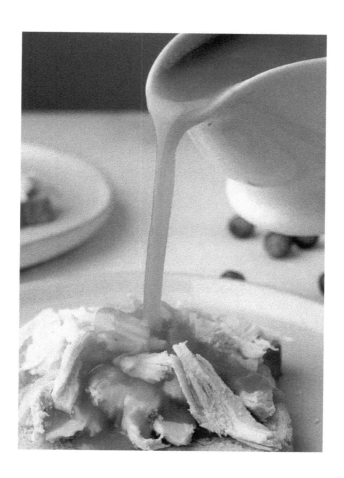

Turmeric Chicken and Veggies

Prep time: 10 minutes I **Cooking time:** 40 minutes I
Servings: 4

Ingredients:

- 1 yellow onion, chopped
- 1 pound chicken breast, skinless, boneless and roughly cubed
- 2 tablespoons olive oil
- 1 cup white mushrooms, sliced
- 1 teaspoon turmeric powder
- 1 cup chicken stock
- 2 garlic cloves, minced
- 2 teaspoons rosemary, chopped
- Salt and black pepper to the tastes
- 1 tablespoon balsamic vinegar
- 1 tablespoon cilantro, chopped

Directions:

1. Heat up a pan with the oil over medium heat, add the onion and the mushrooms and sauté for 10 minutes.
2. Add the meat and brown for 5 minutes more.

3. Add the garlic and the other ingredients, toss, cook over medium heat for 25 minutes more, divide between plates and serve.

Nutrition info per serving: calories 210, fat 5, fiber 8, carbs 15, protein 11

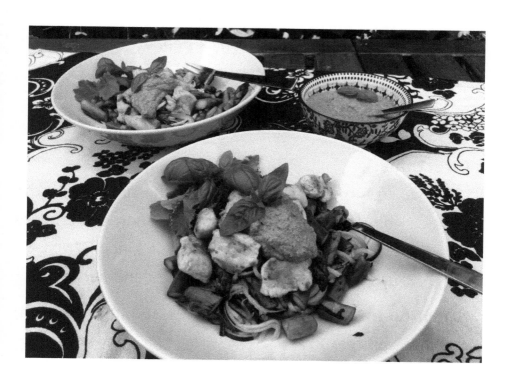

Turkey Roast

Ingredients:

- 2 pounds turkey breast, skinless, boneless and sliced
- 2 tablespoons avocado oil
- 1 yellow onion, sliced
- 2 spring onions, chopped
- A pinch of salt and black pepper
- 1 cup chicken stock
- 2 teaspoons lemon juice
- 1 teaspoon coriander, ground

Directions:

1. In a roasting pan, combine the turkey with the oil, the onion and the other ingredients, toss and bake at 390 degrees F for 1 hour.
2. Divide the mix between plates and serve.

Nutrition info per serving: calories 300, fat 4, fiber 4, carbs 15, protein 27

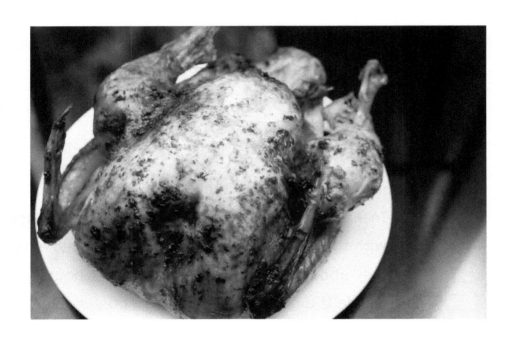

Maple Wings

Prep time: 10 minutes I **Cooking time:** 1 hour I
Servings: 4

Ingredients:

- 2 pounds chicken wings, halved
- 2 tablespoons maple syrup
- A pinch of sea salt and black pepper
- 1 tablespoon apple cider vinegar
- ½ teaspoon thyme, dried
- ½ teaspoon chili powder

Directions:

1. In a roasting pan, combine the chicken wings
   with the maple syrup and the other ingredients,
   toss and bake at 390 degrees F for 1 hour.
2. Divide the mix between plates and serve.

Nutrition info per serving: calories 274, fat 6, fiber 8,
carbs 14, protein 12

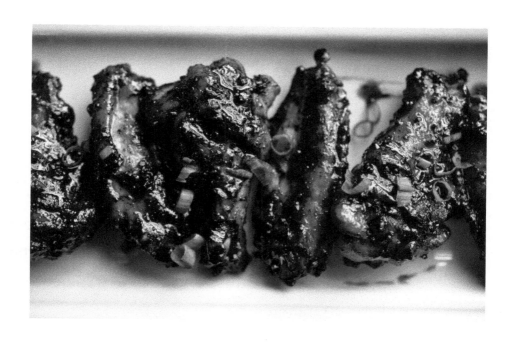

Hot Chicken Wings and Chili Sauce

Prep time: 10 minutes I **Cooking time:** 40 minutes I **Servings:** 4

Ingredients:

- 2 pounds chicken wings, halved
- 2 tablespoons olive oil
- 1 bunch green onions, chopped
- ½ cup chili sauce
- A pinch of salt and black pepper

Directions:

1. Spread the chicken wings on a baking sheet lined with parchment paper, add the oil and the other ingredients, toss and bake at 420 degrees F for 40 minutes.
2. Divide the mix between plates and serve.

Nutrition info per serving: calories 260, fat 4, fiber 2, carbs 12, protein 14

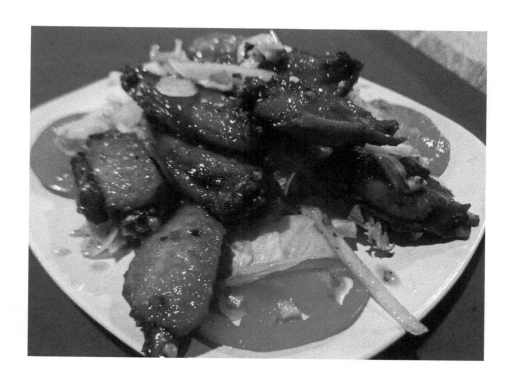

Chicken and Cilantro Sauce

Prep time: 10 minutes I **Cooking time:** 40 minutes I
Servings: 4

Ingredients:

- 1 cup cilantro, chopped
- 1 tablespoon pine nuts, toasted
- ½ cup olive oil
- 1 cup chicken stock
- 4 garlic cloves, minced
- 2 pounds chicken breast, skinless, boneless and sliced
- A pinch of salt and black pepper

Directions:

1. In a blender, combine the cilantro with the pine nuts, the oil and the garlic and pulse well.
2. In a roasting pan, combine the chicken with the cilantro sauce and the remaining ingredients, toss and bake at 390 degrees F for 40 minutes.
3. Divide everything between plates and serve.

Nutrition info per serving: calories 254, fat 3, fiber 3, carbs 7, protein 12

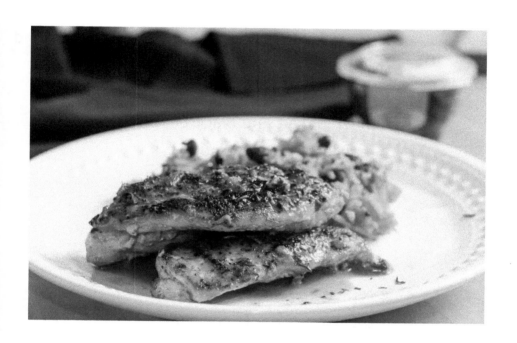

Chicken with Chickpeas

Prep time: 10 minutes I **Cooking time:** 1 hour I
Servings: 4

Ingredients:

- 2 cups chickpeas, cooked
- 2 pounds chicken breast, skinless, boneless and sliced
- 1 cup chicken stock
- A pinch of salt and black pepper
- 1 teaspoon cumin, ground
- 1 teaspoon sweet paprika
- 1 teaspoon coriander, ground
- 2 tablespoons avocado oil
- 1 yellow onion, chopped
- 2 red bell peppers, chopped
- 1 tablespoon garlic powder
- 1 tablespoon chives, chopped

Directions:

1. Heat up a pan with the oil over medium heat, add the onion and the meat and brown for 5 minutes.

2. Add the chickpeas and the other ingredients, toss, introduce in the oven at 350 degrees F, bake for 55 minutes, divide between plates and serve.

Nutrition info per serving: calories 244, fat 11, fiber 4, carbs 10, protein 13

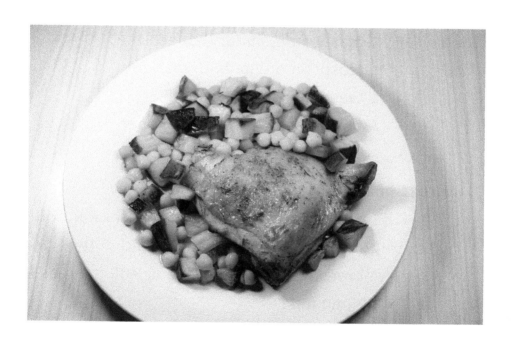

Chicken with Zucchinis

Prep time: 10 minutes I **Cooking time:** 40 minutes I
Servings: 4

Ingredients:

- 2 pounds chicken breasts, skinless, boneless and sliced
- 2 zucchinis, sliced
- 1 cup mushrooms, sliced
- 1 yellow onion, chopped
- 1 teaspoon rosemary, dried
- 1 teaspoon oregano, dried
- 1 teaspoon cumin, ground
- A pinch of salt and black pepper
- 2 tablespoons avocado oil

Directions:

1. In a roasting pan, combine the chicken with the zucchinis, mushrooms and the other ingredients, toss and bake at 400 degrees F for 40 minutes.
2. Divide the mix between plates and serve.

Nutrition info per serving: calories 285, fat 12, fiber 1, carbs 13, protein 16

Chicken and Broccoli

Prep time: 10 minutes I **Cooking time:** 45 minutes I
Servings: 4

Ingredients:

- 2 pounds chicken breasts, skinless, boneless and sliced
- 1 tablespoon olive oil
- 2 tablespoons balsamic vinegar
- ½ pound broccoli florets
- 2 tablespoons coconut aminos
- 2 garlic cloves, minced
- 3 green onions, chopped

Directions:

1. In a roasting pan, combine the chicken with the oil, the vinegar and the other ingredients, toss and bake at 400 degrees F for 45 minutes.
2. Divide the mix between plates and serve.

Nutrition info per serving: calories 250, fat 4, fiber 5, carbs 10, protein 12

Chicken with Coconut Corn

Prep time: 10 minutes I **Cooking time:** 8 hours I
Servings: 6

Ingredients:

- 2 pounds chicken breast, skinless, boneless and sliced
- 2 tablespoons olive oil
- 2 cups corn
- 2 teaspoons garlic powder
- A pinch of salt and black pepper
- 2 cups coconut milk
- 2 tablespoons parsley, chopped
- 3 green onions, chopped

Directions:

1. In your slow cooker, combine the chicken with the oil, the corn and the other ingredients, toss, put the lid on and cook on Low for 8 hours.
2. Divide everything between plates and serve.

Nutrition info per serving: calories 265, fat 8, fiber 10, carbs 10, protein 24

Chicken and Fennel Mix

Prep time: 10 minutes I **Cooking time:** 45 minutes I
Servings: 4

Ingredients:

- 2 yellow onions, chopped
- 2 pounds chicken breast, skinless, boneless and roughly cubed
- 2 fennel bulbs, shredded
- 4 garlic cloves, minced
- 2 tablespoons olive oil
- 1 cup chicken stock
- A pinch of sea salt and black pepper
- 2 tablespoons parsley, chopped

Directions:

1. Heat up a pan with the oil over medium heat, add the onions and the garlic and sauté for 5 minutes.
2. Add the fennel and the meat and brown for 5 minutes more.
3. Add the rest of the ingredients, toss, bring to a simmer and cook over medium heat for 35 minutes.
4. Divide everything between plates and serve.

Nutrition info per serving: calories 200, fat 4, fiber 4, carbs 10, protein 16

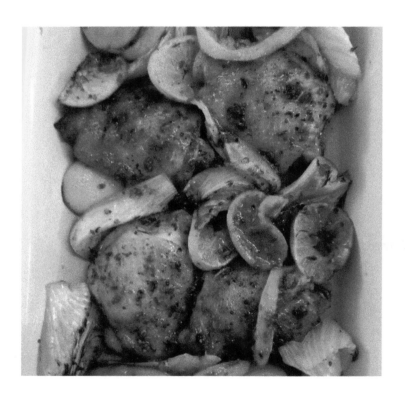

Duck with Green Beans

Prep time: 10 minutes I **Cooking time:** 40 minutes I
Servings: 4

Ingredients:

- 2 pounds duck legs, skinless, boneless and cubed
- 4 scallions, chopped
- 2 tablespoons olive oil
- 1 pound green beans, trimmed and halved
- 1 tablespoon pine nuts, chipped
- 2 tablespoons parsley, chopped
- 2 tablespoons tomato puree
- A pinch of salt and black pepper

Directions:

1. Heat up a pan with the oil over medium heat, add the scallions and the meat and brown for 5 minutes.
2. Add the green beans and the other ingredients, toss, cook over medium heat for 35 minutes more, divide between plates and serve.

Nutrition info per serving: calories 522, fat 22.2, fiber 4.6, carbs 10.3, protein 68.8

Indian Chicken Mix

Prep time: 10 minutes I **Cooking time:** 40 minutes I
Servings: 4

Ingredients:

- 1 pound chicken breasts, skinless, boneless and cubed
- 1 yellow onion, chopped
- 2 tablespoons olive oil
- 1 tablespoon garam masala
- ½ teaspoon ginger, grated
- ½ teaspoon cumin, ground
- 1 teaspoon turmeric, ground
- A pinch of salt and black pepper
- 2 cups coconut milk
- 1 tablespoon coriander, chopped

Directions:

1. Heat up a pan with the oil over medium-high heat, add the onion and the ginger and sauté for 5 minutes.
2. Add the meat and brown for 5 minutes more.
3. Add the garam masala and the other ingredients, toss, bring to a simmer, cook over

medium heat for 30 minutes more, divide between plates and serve.

Nutrition info per serving: calories 566, fat 44.2, fiber 3.4, carbs 9.9, protein 36

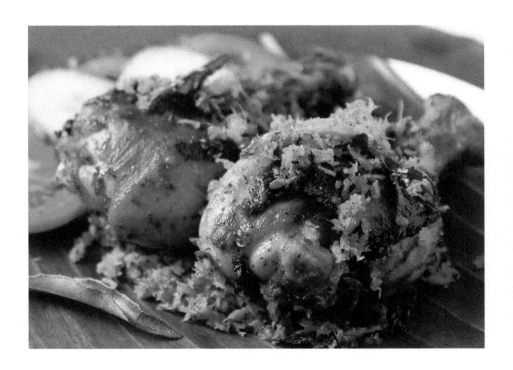

Duck with Kale

Prep time: 10 minutes I **Cooking time:** 35 minutes I
Servings: 4

Ingredients:

- 1 yellow onion, chopped
- 2 garlic cloves, minced
- 2 tablespoons olive oil
- 1 teaspoon oregano, dried
- 2 pounds duck breast, skinless, boneless and cut into strips
- 1 cup chicken stock
- 2 cups kale, torn
- Juice of 1 lime
- A pinch of salt and black pepper
- 1 cup tomatoes, chopped
- 1 teaspoon sweet paprika
- 3 tablespoons cilantro, chopped

Directions:

1. Heat up a pan with the oil over medium heat, add the onion and the garlic and sauté for 5 minutes.
2. Add the duck and brown for 5 minutes more.

3. Add the oregano and the other ingredients, toss, cook over medium heat for 25 minutes more.

4. Divide the mix between plates and serve.

Nutrition info per serving: calories 470, fat 9.3, fiber 3, carbs 12, protein 11

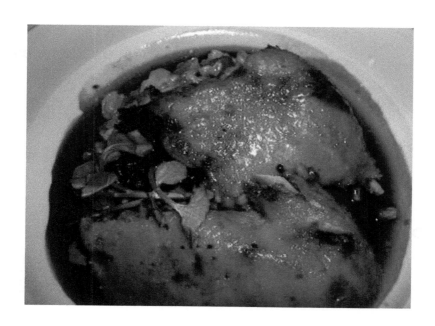

Chicken with Spinach Mix

Prep time: 10 minutes I **Cooking time:** 40 minutes I
Servings: 4

Ingredients:

- 1 yellow onion, chopped
- 5 garlic cloves, minced
- 1 tablespoon orange juice
- 2 tablespoons olive oil
- 1 tablespoon orange zest, grated
- 1 cup chicken stock
- 1 pound chicken breast, skinless, boneless and cubed
- A pinch of salt and black pepper
- 1 cup baby spinach
- 1 teaspoon cumin, ground
- 1 tablespoon cilantro, chopped

Directions:

1. Heat up a pan with the oil over medium heat, add the onion and the garlic and sauté for 5 minutes.
2. Add the meat, orange juice and zest and brown for 5 minutes more.

3. Add the rest of the ingredients, toss, cook over medium heat for 30 minutes, divide between plates and serve.

Nutrition info per serving: calories 250, fat 3, fiber 3, carbs 14, protein 7

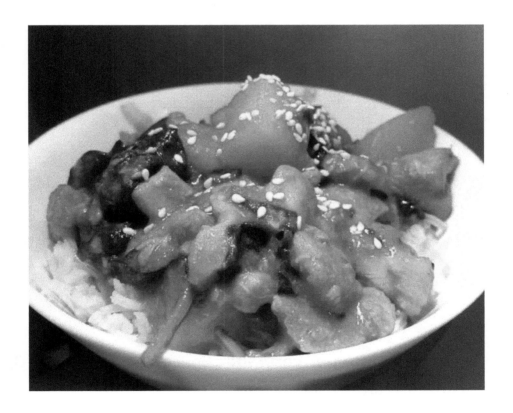

Thyme Turkey

Prep time: 10 minutes I **Cooking time:** 8 hours I
Servings: 4

Ingredients:

- 2 tablespoons olive oil
- 1 yellow onion, chopped
- 2 pounds turkey breast, skinless, boneless and cubed
- 1 cup chicken stock
- 1 teaspoon sweet paprika
- 1 teaspoon chili powder
- 1 tablespoon thyme, chopped
- A pinch of salt and black pepper

Directions:

1. In a slow cooker, combine the onion with the meat, the oil and the other ingredients, toss, put the lid on and cook on Low for 8 hours.
2. Divide the mix between plates and serve.

Nutrition info per serving: calories 200, fat 5, fiber 3, carbs 14, protein 11

Turkey with Zoodles

Prep time: 10 minutes I **Cooking time:** 30 minutes I
Servings: 4

Ingredients:

- 1 yellow onion, chopped
- 1 tablespoon olive oil
- 1 pound turkey breast, skinless, boneless and cut into strips
- Salt and black pepper to the taste
- 1 tablespoon parsley, chopped
- Juice of 1 lime
- 2 zucchinis, cut with a spiralizer
- 1 cup tomatoes, cubed
- 1 tablespoon chives, chopped

Directions:

1. Heat up a pan with the oil over medium-high heat, add the onion and the meat and brown for 5 minutes.
2. Add the zucchini noodles and the other ingredients, toss, cook over medium heat for 25 minutes more, divide between plates and serve.

Nutrition info per serving: calories 180, fat 4, fiber 8, carbs 11, protein 10

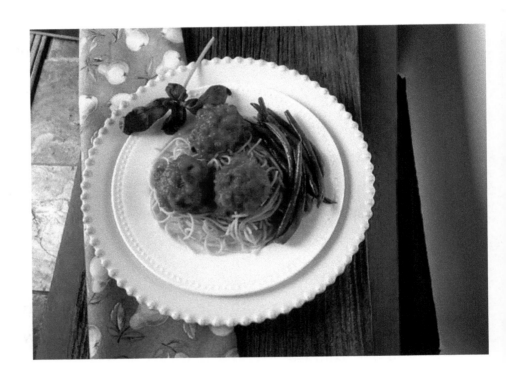

Turkey with Rosemary Cabbage

Prep time: 10 minutes I **Cooking time:** 40 minutes I
Servings: 4

Ingredients:

- 1 pound turkey breast, skinless, boneless and cubed
- 1 yellow onion, chopped
- 1 tablespoon sweet paprika
- 3 cups cabbage, shredded
- ½ cup chicken stock
- Salt and black pepper to the taste
- ¼ teaspoon garlic powder
- ½ teaspoon rosemary, dried

Directions:

1. Heat up a pan with the oil over medium heat, add the onion and the meat and brown for 5 minutes.
2. Add the cabbage and the other ingredients, toss, cook over medium heat for 35 minutes more, divide between plates and serve.

Nutrition info per serving: calories 240, fat 15, fiber 1, carbs 9, protein 15

Chicken with Coconut Beets

Prep time: 10 minutes I **Cooking time:** 45 minutes I
Servings: 4

Ingredients:

- 2 pounds chicken breasts, boneless, skinless
  and sliced
- 4 scallions, chopped
- 2 spring onions, chopped
- 2 beets, peeled and cubed
- 2 tablespoons olive oil
- 1 cup coconut cream
- Salt and black pepper to the taste
- 2 garlic cloves, minced

Directions:

1. In a roasting pan, combine the chicken with the
   scallions and the other ingredients, toss, and
   bake at 400 degrees F for 45 minutes.
2. Divide everything between plates and serve.

Nutrition info per serving: calories 255, fat 10, fiber
5, carbs 12, protein 20

Chicken with Mixed Veggies

Prep time: 10 minutes I **Cooking time:** 45 minutes I
Servings: 4

Ingredients:

- 2 pounds chicken breast, skinless, boneless and sliced
- 1 bunch asparagus, trimmed and halved
- 1 cup green beans, trimmed and halved
- 2 tablespoons avocado oil
- 1 yellow onion, chopped
- 1 cup chicken stock
- A pinch of salt and black pepper
- 1 tablespoon cilantro, chopped

Directions:

1. Heat up a pan with the oil over medium heat, add the onion and sauté for 5 minutes.
2. Add the meat and brown for 5 minutes more.
3. Add the rest of the ingredients, toss, introduce in the oven and bake at 380 degrees F for 35 minutes.
4. Divide everything between plates and serve.

Nutrition info per serving: calories 500, fat 27, fiber 3, carbs 4, protein 47

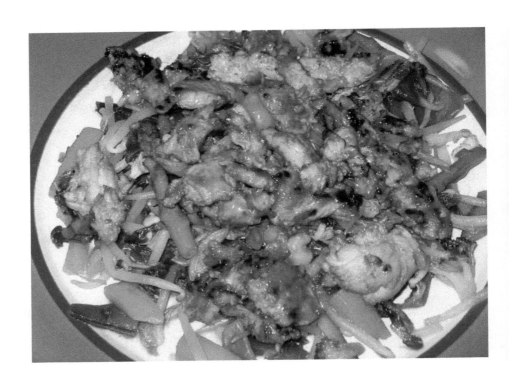

Chicken Salad

Prep time: 10 minutes I **Cooking time:** 0 minutes I
Servings: 4

Ingredients:

- 2 cups rotisserie chicken, cooked and shredded
- 1 cup tomatoes, cubed
- 1 cucumber, sliced
- 1 yellow onion, chopped
- 2 tablespoons olive oil
- 1 tablespoon lemon juice
- Salt and black pepper to the taste
- 1 tablespoon chives, chopped

Directions:

1. In a salad bowl, combine the chicken with the tomatoes, the cucumber and the other ingredients, toss and serve.

Nutrition info per serving: calories 234, fat 8, fiber 4, carbs 12, protein 15

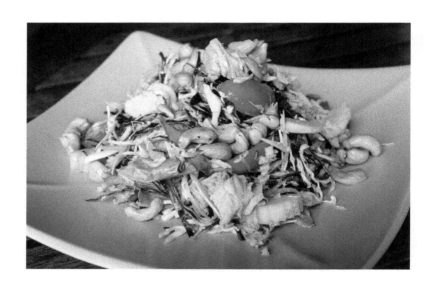

Turkey and Radish Salad

Prep time: 10 minutes I **Cooking time:** 25 minutes I
Servings: 4

Ingredients:

- 4 spring onions, chopped
- 1 pound turkey breast, skinless, boneless and cut into strips
- 2 tablespoons olive oil
- 1 cup radishes, cubed
- 1 tablespoon balsamic vinegar
- ½ cup baby spinach
- 2 tablespoons parsley, chopped
- A pinch of salt and black pepper

Directions:

1. Heat up a pan with the oil over medium heat, add the spring onions and the turkey meat and brown for 5 minutes.
2. Add the rest of the ingredients, toss, cook over medium heat for 20 minutes, divide into bowls and serve.

Nutrition info per serving: calories 190, fat 9, fiber 1.6, carbs 7.2, protein 20

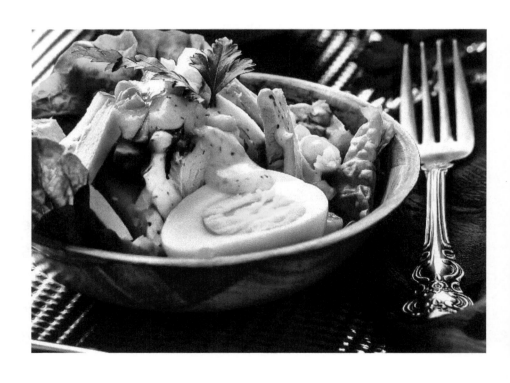

Chicken with Sweet Onions

Prep time: 10 minutes I **Cooking time:** 40 minutes I
Servings: 4

Ingredients:

- 2 pounds chicken breasts, skinless, boneless and sliced
- 2 tablespoons olive oil
- Salt and black pepper to the taste
- 2 tablespoons balsamic vinegar
- 2 sweet onions, sliced
- 2 garlic cloves, minced
- 1 teaspoon Italian seasoning
- 1 teaspoon red pepper flakes

Directions:

1. Heat up a pan with the oil over medium heat, add the onions and the meat and brown for 10 minutes.
2. Add the vinegar and the other ingredients, toss, bring to a simmer and cook over medium heat for 30 minutes more.
3. Divide the mix between plates and serve.

Nutrition info per serving: calories 522, fat 24.3, fiber 1.3, carbs 6.1, protein 66.4

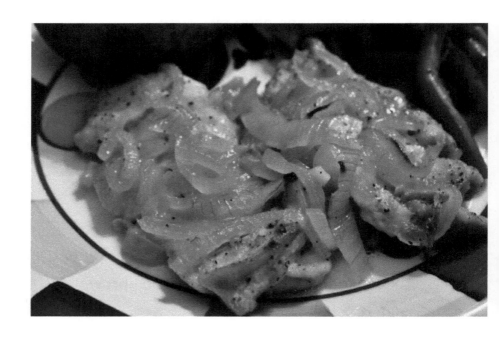

Turkey and Mozzarella Artichokes Mix

Prep time: 5 minutes I **Cooking time:** 25 minutes I **Servings:** 4

Ingredients:

- 2 tablespoons olive oil
- 1 turkey breast, skinless, boneless and sliced
- A pinch of black pepper
- 1 tablespoon basil, chopped
- 3 garlic cloves, minced
- 14 ounces artichokes, chopped
- 1 cup coconut cream
- ¾ cup mozzarella, shredded

Directions:

1. Heat up a pan with the oil over medium-high heat, add the meat, garlic and the black pepper, toss and cook for 5 minutes.
2. Add the rest of the ingredients except the cheese, toss and cook over medium heat for 15 minutes.
3. Sprinkle the cheese, cook everything for 5 minutes more, divide between plates and serve.

Nutrition info per serving: calories 300, fat 22.2, fiber 7.2, carbs 16.5, protein 13.6

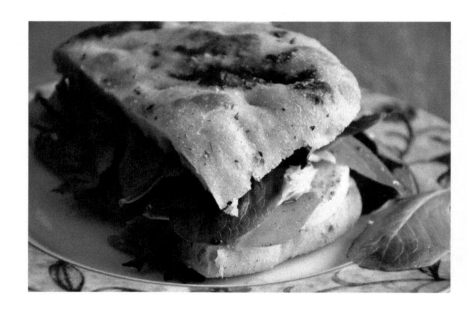

Oregano and Chives Turkey Mix

Prep time: 10 minutes I **Cooking time:** 30 minutes I
Servings: 4

Ingredients:

- 2 tablespoons avocado oil
- 1 red onion, chopped
- 2 garlic cloves, minced
- A pinch of black pepper
- 1 tablespoon oregano, chopped
- 1 big turkey breast, skinless, boneless and cubed
- 1 and ½ cups beef stock
- 1 tablespoon chives, chopped

Directions:

1. Heat up a pan with the oil over medium heat, add the onion, stir and sauté for 3 minutes.
2. Add the garlic and the meat, toss and cook for 3 minutes more.
3. Add the rest of the ingredients, toss, simmer everything over medium heat fro 25 minutes, divide between plates and serve.

Nutrition info per serving: calories 76, fat 2.1, fiber 1.7, carbs 6.4, protein 8.3

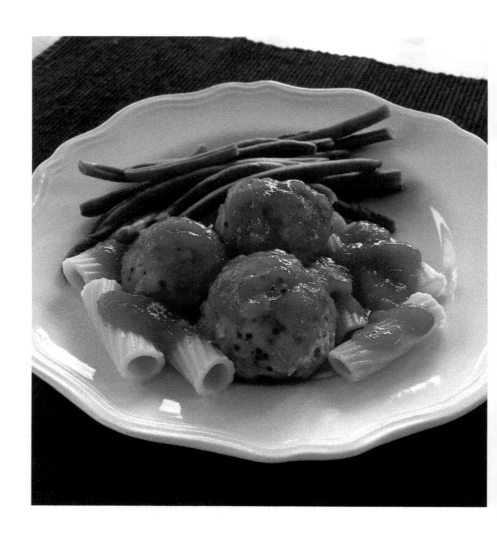

Orange Balsamic Chicken

Prep time: 10 minutes I **Cooking time:** 35 minutes I
Servings: 4

Ingredients:

- 1 tablespoon avocado oil
- 1 pound chicken breast, skinless, boneless and halved
- 2 garlic cloves, minced
- 2 shallots, chopped
- ½ cup orange juice
- 1 tablespoon orange zest, grated
- 3 tablespoons balsamic vinegar
- 1 teaspoon rosemary, chopped

Directions:

1. Heat up a pan with the oil over medium-high heat, add the shallots and the garlic, toss and sauté for 2 minutes.
2. Add the meat, toss gently and cook for 3 minutes more.
3. Add the rest of the ingredients, toss, introduce the pan in the oven and bake at 340 degrees F for 30 minutes.

4. Divide between plates and serve.

Nutrition info per serving: calories 159, fat 3.4, fiber 0.5, carbs 5.4, protein 24.6

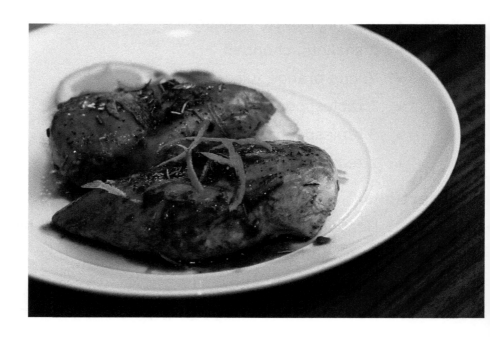

Garlic Turkey

Prep time: 10 minutes I **Cooking time:** 40 minutes I
Servings: 4

Ingredients:

- 1 turkey breast, boneless, skinless and cubed
- ½ pound white mushrooms, halved
- 1/3 cup coconut aminos
- 2 garlic cloves, minced
- 2 tablespoons olive oil
- A pinch of black pepper
- 2 green onion, chopped
- 3 tablespoons garlic sauce
- 1 tablespoon rosemary, chopped

Directions:

1. Heat up a pan with the oil over medium heat, add the green onions, garlic sauce and the garlic and sauté for 5 minutes.
2. Add the meat and brown it for 5 minutes more.
3. Add the rest of the ingredients, introduce in the oven and bake at 390 degrees F for 30 minutes.
4. Divide the mix between plates and serve.

Nutrition info per serving: calories 154, fat 8.1, fiber 1.5, carbs 11.5, protein 9.8

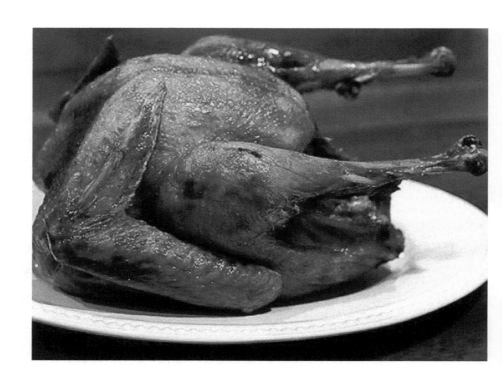

Chicken and Kalamata Olives

Prep time: 10 minutes I **Cooking time:** 25 minutes I
Servings: 4

Ingredients:

- 1 pound chicken breasts, skinless, boneless and roughly cubed
- A pinch of black pepper
- 1 tablespoon avocado oil
- 1 red onion, chopped
- 1 cup coconut milk
- 1 tablespoon lemon juice
- 1 cup kalamata olives, pitted and sliced
- ¼ cup cilantro, chopped

Directions:

1. Heat up a pan with the oil over medium-high heat, add the onion and the meat and brown for 5 minutes.
2. Add the rest of the ingredients, toss, bring to a simmer and cook over medium heat for 20 minutes more.
3. Divide between plates and serve.

Nutrition info per serving: calories 409, fat 26.8, fiber 3.2, carbs 8.3, protein 34.9

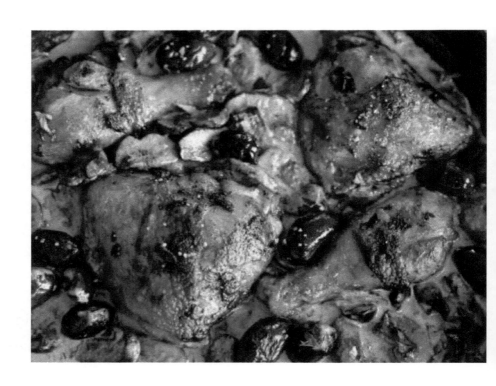

Balsamic Turkey

Prep time: 10 minutes I **Cooking time:** 25 minutes I
Servings: 4

Ingredients:

- 1 tablespoon avocado oil
- 1 turkey breast, skinless, boneless and sliced
- A pinch of black pepper
- 1 yellow onion, chopped
- 4 peaches, stones removed and cut into wedges
- ¼ cup balsamic vinegar
- 2 tablespoons chives, chopped

Directions:

1. Heat up a pan with the oil over medium-high heat, add the meat and the onion, toss and brown for 5 minutes.
2. Add the rest of the ingredients except the chives, toss gently and bake at 390 degrees F for 20 minutes.
3. Divide everything between plates and serve with the chives sprinkled on top.

Nutrition info per serving: calories 123, fat 1.6, fiber 3.3, carbs 18.8, protein 9.1

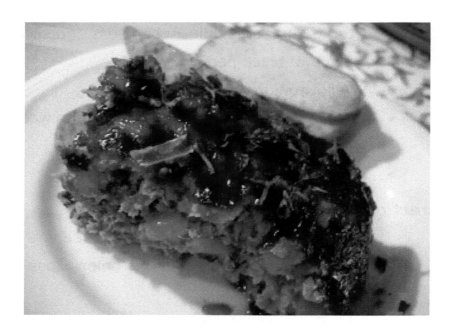

Coconut Basil Chicken and Greens

Prep time: 10 minutes I **Cooking time:** 25 minutes I
Servings: 4

Ingredients:

- 1 tablespoon avocado oil
- 1 pound chicken breast, skinless, boneless and cubed
- ½ teaspoon basil, dried
- A pinch of black pepper
- ¼ cup veggie stock
- 2 cups baby spinach
- 2 shallots, chopped
- 2 garlic cloves, minced
- ½ teaspoon sweet paprika
- 2/3 cup coconut cream
- 2 tablespoons cilantro, chopped

Directions:

1. Heat up a pan with the oil over medium-high heat, add the meat, basil, black pepper and brown for 5 minutes.
2. Add the shallots and the garlic and cook for another 5 minutes.

89

3. Add the rest of the ingredients, toss, bring to a simmer and cook over medium heat fro 15 minutes more.
4. Divide between plates and serve hot.

Nutrition info per serving: calories 237, fat 12.9, fiber 1.6, carbs 4.7, protein 25.8

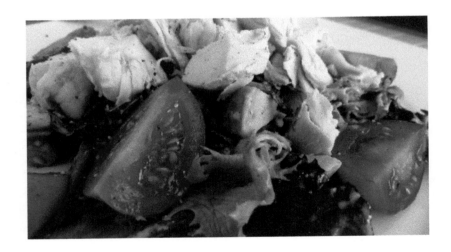

Paprika Chicken and Asparagus

Prep time: 10 minutes I **Cooking time:** 25 minutes I
Servings: 4

Ingredients:

- 2 chicken breasts, skinless, boneless and cubed
- 2 tablespoons avocado oil
- 2 spring onions, chopped
- 1 bunch asparagus, trimmed and halved
- ½ teaspoon sweet paprika
- A pinch of black pepper
- 14 ounces tomatoes, chopped

Directions:

1. Heat up a pan with the oil over medium-high heat, add the meat and the spring onions, stir and cook for 5 minutes.
2. Add the asparagus and the other ingredients, toss, cover the pan and cook over medium heat for 20 minutes.
3. Divide everything between plates and serve.

Nutrition info per serving: calories 171, fat 6.4, fiber 2,6, carbs 6.4, protein 22.2

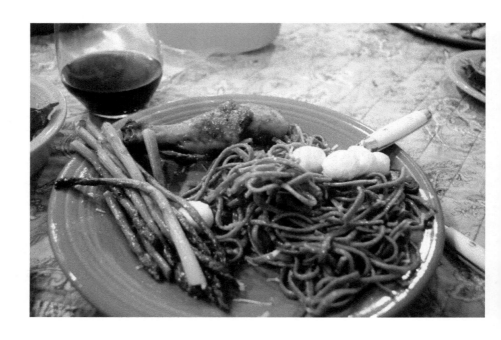

Turkey and Creamy Sauce

Prep time: 10 minutes I **Cooking time:** 25 minutes I
Servings: 4

Ingredients:

- 1 tablespoon olive oil
- 1 big turkey breast, skinless, boneless and cubed
- 2 cups broccoli florets
- 2 shallots, chopped
- 2 garlic cloves, minced
- 1 tablespoon basil, chopped
- 1 tablespoon cilantro, chopped
- ½ cup coconut cream

Directions:

1. Heat up a pan with the oil over medium-high heat, add the meat, shallots and the garlic, toss and brown for 5 minutes.
2. Add the broccoli and the other ingredients, toss everything, cook for 20 minutes over medium heat, divide between plates and serve.

Nutrition info per serving: calories 165, fat 11.5, fiber 2.1, carbs 7.9, protein 9.6

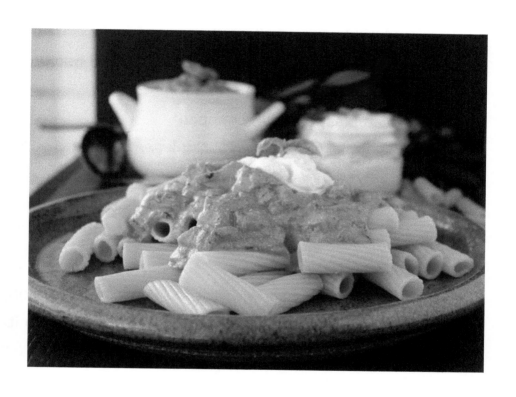

Chicken and Dill Veggies Mix

Prep time: 10 minutes I **Cooking time:** 25 minutes I
Servings: 4

Ingredients:

- 2 tablespoons olive oil
- 10 ounces green beans, trimmed and halved
- 1 yellow onion, chopped
- 1 tablespoon dill, chopped
- 2 chicken breasts, skinless, boneless and halved
- 2 cups tomato sauce
- ½ teaspoon red pepper flakes, crushed

Directions:

1. Heat up a pan with the oil over medium-high heat, add the onion and the meat and brown it for 2 minutes on each side.
2. Add the green beans and the other ingredients, toss, introduce in the oven and bake at 380 degrees F fro 20 minutes.
3. Divide between plates and serve right away.

Nutrition info per serving: calories 391, fat 17.8, fiber 5, carbs 14.8, protein 43.9

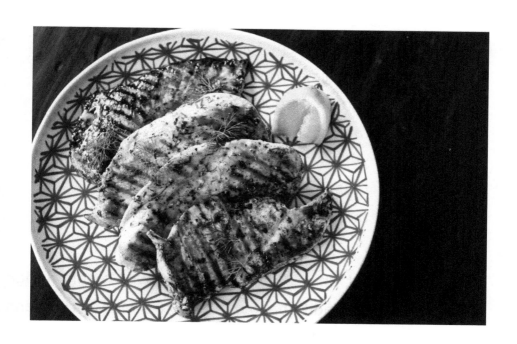

Chicken with Mushrooms and Zucchini

Prep time: 5 minutes I **Cooking time:** 25 minutes I
Servings: 4

Ingredients:

- 1 pound chicken breasts, skinless, boneless and cubed
- 1 cup chicken stock
- 2 zucchinis, roughly cubed
- 1 cup mushrooms, halved
- 1 tablespoon olive oil
- 1 yellow onion, chopped
- 1 teaspoon chili powder
- 1 tablespoon cilantro, chopped

Directions:

1. Heat up a pan with the oil over medium-high heat, add the meat and the onion, toss and brown for 5 minutes.
2. Add the zucchinis and the rest of the ingredients, toss gently, reduce the heat to medium and cook for 20 minutes.
3. Divide everything between plates and serve.

Nutrition info per serving: calories 284, fat 12.3, fiber 2.4, carbs 8, protein 35

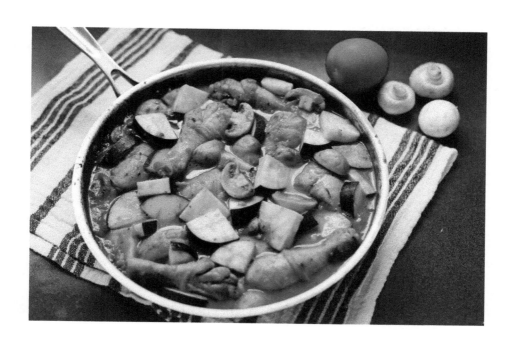

Avocado and Garlic Chicken Mix

Prep time: 10 minutes I **Cooking time:** 20 minutes I
Servings: 4

Ingredients:

- 2 chicken breasts, skinless, boneless and halved
- Juice of ½ lemon
- 2 tablespoons olive oil
- 2 garlic cloves, minced
- ½ cup veggie stock
- 1 avocado, peeled, pitted and cut into wedges
- A pinch of black pepper

Directions:

1. Heat up a pan with the oil over medium heat, add the garlic and the meat and brown for 2 minutes on each side.
2. Add the lemon juice and the other ingredients, bring to a simmer and cook over medium heat fro 15 minutes.
3. Divide the whole mix between plates and serve.

Nutrition info per serving: calories 436, fat 27.3, fiber 3.6, carbs 5.6, protein 41.8

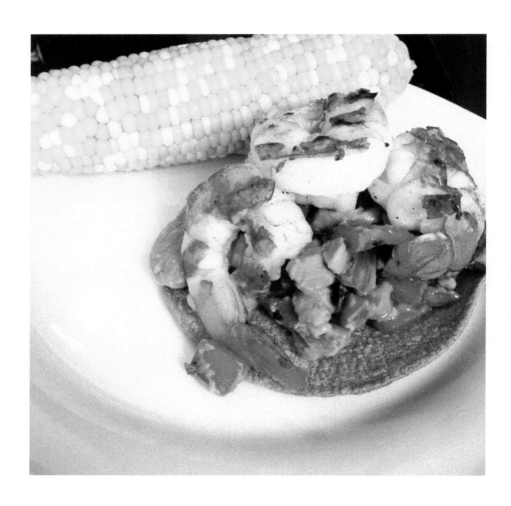

Turkey and Ginger Baby Spinach

Prep time: 10 minutes I **Cooking time:** 20 minutes I
Servings: 4

Ingredients:

- 1 turkey breast, boneless, skinless and roughly cubed
- 2 scallions, chopped
- 1 pound baby spinach
- 2 tablespoons olive oil
- ½ teaspoon ginger, grated
- A pinch of black pepper
- ½ cup veggie stock

Directions:

1. Heat up a pot with the oil over medium-high heat, add the scallions and the ginger and sauté for 2 minutes.
2. Add the meat and brown for 5 minutes more.
3. Add the rest of the ingredients, toss, simmer for 13 minutes more, divide between plates and serve.

Nutrition info per serving: calories 125, fat 8, fiber 1.7, carbs 5.5, protein 9.3

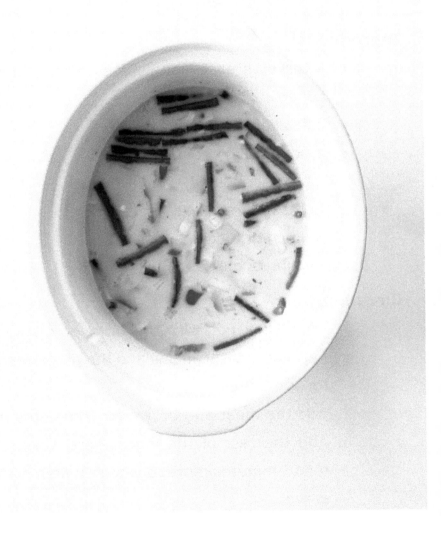

Chicken with Cilantro Red Onion Mix

Prep time: 10 minutes I **Cooking time:** 25 minutes I
Servings: 4

Ingredients:

- 2 chicken breasts, skinless, boneless and roughly cubed
- 3 red onions, sliced
- 2 tablespoons olive oil
- 1 cup veggie stock
- A pinch of black pepper
- 1 tablespoon cilantro, chopped
- 1 tablespoon chives, chopped

Directions:

1. Heat up a pan with the oil over medium heat, add the onions and a pinch of black pepper, and sauté for 10 minutes stirring often.
2. Add the chicken and cook for 3 minutes more.
3. Add the rest of the ingredients, bring to a simmer and cook over medium heat for 12 minutes more.
4. Divide the chicken and onions mix between plates and serve.

Nutrition info per serving : calories 364, fat 17.5, fiber 2.1, carbs 8.8, protein 41.7

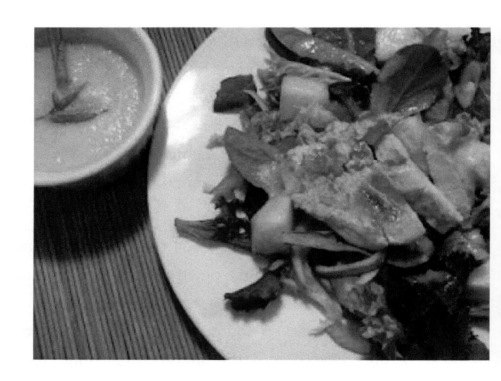

Turkey and Serrano Rice

Prep time: 10 minutes I **Cooking time:** 42 minutes I
Servings: 4

Ingredients:

- 1 turkey breast, skinless, boneless and cubed
- 1 cup brown rice
- 2 cups veggie stock
- 1 teaspoon hot paprika
- 2 small Serrano peppers, chopped
- 2 garlic cloves, minced
- 2 tablespoons olive oil
- ½ red bell pepper chopped
- A pinch of black pepper

Directions:

1. Heat up a pan with the oil over medium heat, add the Serrano peppers and garlic and sauté for 2 minutes.
2. Add the meat and brown it for 5 minutes.
3. Add the rice and the other ingredients, bring to a simmer and cook over medium heat for 35 minutes.
4. Stir, divide between plates and serve.

Nutrition info per serving: calories 271, fat 7.7, fiber 1.7, carbs 42, protein 7.8

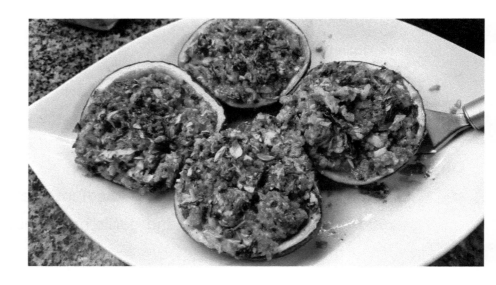

Chicken and Leeks

Prep time: 10 minutes I **Cooking time:** 40 minutes I
Servings: 4

Ingredients:

- 1 pound chicken breast, skinless, boneless and cubed
- A pinch of black pepper
- 2 tablespoons avocado oil
- 1 tablespoon tomato sauce
- 1 cup veggie stock
- 4 leek, roughly chopped
- ½ cup lemon juice

Directions:

1. Heat up a pan with the oil over medium heat, add the leeks, toss and sauté for 10 minutes.
2. Add the chicken and the other ingredients, toss, cook over medium heat for 20 minutes more, divide between plates and serve.

Nutrition info per serving : calories 199, fat 13.3, fiber 5, carbs 7.6, protein 17.4

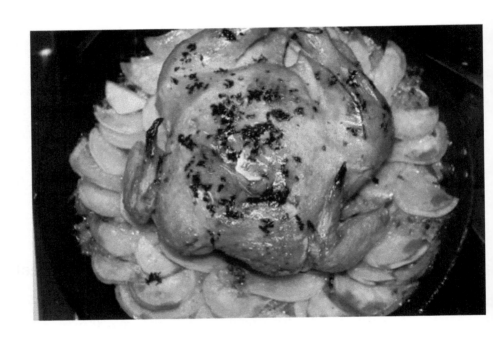

Lightning Source UK Ltd.
Milton Keynes UK
UKHW020801110621
385329UK00001B/146